YOUR KNOWLEDGE HAS VALUE

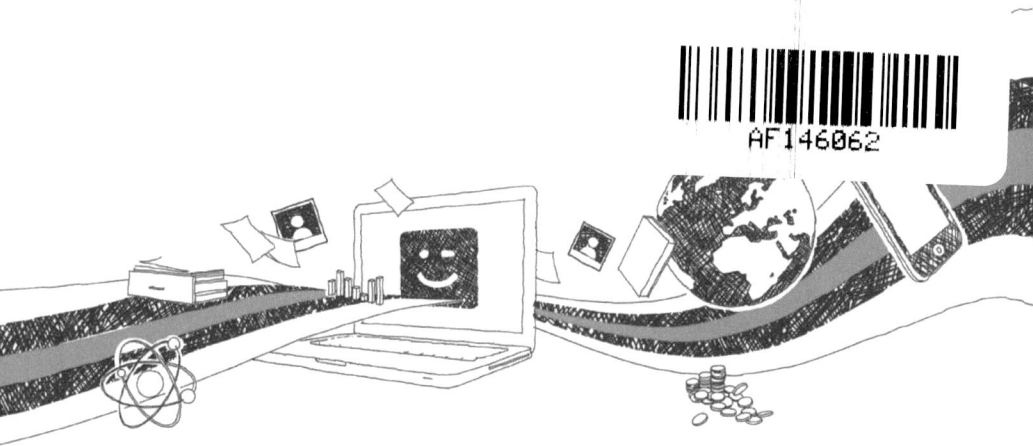

- We will publish your bachelor's and master's thesis, essays and papers

- Your own eBook and book - sold worldwide in all relevant shops

- Earn money with each sale

Upload your text at www.GRIN.com
and publish for free

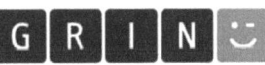

Bibliographic information published by the German National Library:

The German National Library lists this publication in the National Bibliography; detailed bibliographic data are available on the Internet at http://dnb.dnb.de .

Imprint:

Copyright © 2015 GRIN Verlag, Open Publishing GmbH
Print and binding: Books on Demand GmbH, Norderstedt Germany
ISBN: 978-3-668-02401-4

This book at GRIN:

http://www.grin.com/en/e-book/304003/male-invovlement-in-their-partner-s-pregnancy-and-childbirth

Vijeyata Naidu

Male invovlement in their partner's pregnancy and childbirth

An exploratory study in Bilaspur district of Chhattisgarh, India

GRIN Publishing

GRIN - Your knowledge has value

Since its foundation in 1998, GRIN has specialized in publishing academic texts by students, college teachers and other academics as e-book and printed book. The website www.grin.com is an ideal platform for presenting term papers, final papers, scientific essays, dissertations and specialist books.

Visit us on the internet:

http://www.grin.com/

http://www.facebook.com/grincom

http://www.twitter.com/grin_com

"Male involvement in their partner's pregnancy and childbirth; An Exploratory study in the Bilaspur district of Chhattisgarh state"

By

P Vijeyata Naidu

A Thesis

Submitted to the School of Medical Sciences

in Partial Fulfillment of the Requirements for

the Degree of Masters in Public health

at the University of Hyderabad

Hyderabad Central University, Hyderabad, India

2015

ACKNOWLEDGEMENT

The writing of this dissertation has been one of the most significant academic challenges I have ever had to face. I think it would be an appropriate analogy if I would call it a 'journey'. This dissertation has taught me various aspects of research and ways to deal with respondents in the real world. Without the support, patience and guidance of the following people, this study would not have been completed. It is to them that I owe my deepest gratitude.

Foremost, I would like to express my sincere gratitude to my advisor and supervisor Dr B.R Shammana for the continuous support of my study and research, for his patience, motivation, enthusiasm, and immense knowledge. His guidance helped me all the time

In my research and writing of this thesis. I could not have imagined having a better advisor and mentor for my study.

I am also grateful to my co –supervisor 1 in the study, Mr Jagannath Kompella, whose selfless time and care were sometimes all that kept me going,I am extremely thankful and indebted to him for sharing his expertise, sincere and valuable guidance and encouragement extended to me.

I would also like to take up this opportunity to thank my co-supervisor 2 professor Nandkishore Kannuri , who has helped me to narrow down to this particular topic and encouraged me to take it up as my dissertation work.

I would like to thank Miss Soniya Jaiswal , a field worker and a very good friend for her guidance and support while conducting the interviews in various Anganwadi centres of Bilaspur.

Last but not the least I thank my family and friends to be extremely supportive and encouraging towards me. I dedicate the study to all those who have helped me in the completion of the study and also to those who participated in the study. Because it is their participation and willingness to come and volunteer for the interviews, which has made this study a reality.

Table of Contents

Key terms

- Mitanin: Mitanins are the community health volunteers (otherwise known as ASHA in other states) Over 72,000 such volunteers are working in Chhattisgarh hamlet wise called as 'Mitanin' with literal meaning as 'female friend'. These women voluntarily increase the community demand for modern medical care and help the government in ensuring percolation of health programmes at grass-root level.

- ANM: ANM stands for 'Auxiliary Nurse Midwife' . ANM is considered as lowest line agency of health department at Panchayat level and the first point of contact between needs and services, between people and organization. They are the person who are in charge of Sub health centre.

- AWW: AWW stands for ' Anganwadi worker'. The integrated child development services comprises of Anganwadi workers. Their responsibility is to manage the Anganwadi centres and promote its services for the children from the age group of 4 to 6 years and also make registration of pregnant women at the community level.

- BCC: Behaviour change and communications strategies.

- IEC: Information, education and communication strategies.

EXECUTIVE SUMMARY

Male involvement has shown to yield positive results in the health of the women and their children, according to many studies conducted earlier in India and Abroad. This study thus subscribes to the hypothesis that interventions that include men during pregnancy and childbirth has greater and positive impact on maternal and child health. Taking references from similar studies which assessed male involvement in either qualitative or quantitative fashion, this utilizes mixed methods wherein the quantitative data and qualitative data were collected concurrently to understand Male involvement in terms of Awareness levels, reproductive health patterns, preferences and perception regarding the health care services available, factors influencing health services seeking behaviour, male partner's support during all the significant events during pregnancy, delivery and childcare, financial and emotional support from the male partner, assistance obtained from Mitanins, Auxillary nurse midwives, Anganwadi workers, Doctors, and assistance derived from the social network, i.e Neighbours and family members.

The location selected for the study is Bilaspur district of Chhattisgarh India. It hosts a population size of 2,663,629 according to the 2011 census. It is the second largest city after the capital city if Raipur in the entire state and governs around 1635 villages. Bilaspur served as an ideal location as it serves a huge diversity of population within the district. The study took an exploratory approach and adapted mixed methods comprising of questionnaire interviews with 50 couples belonging to 4 different locations in Bilaspur.

The locations were selected according to convenience and the sampling method used was random stratified sampling wherein the sample was broken into small strata and at the same time capturing maximum variation. The selection criteria was to interview only those couples who were expecting a baby at the time of the interviews and couples who are parents of at least one child of 2 years or less.

The tools used for undertaking the study includes personal interaction questionnaire, Focus group discussion and key informant interviews along with reference secondary information collected for the purpose.

The significant observations made from the study suggests that there is maximum involvement of husband in most of the cases and the outcome has been encouraging.

In cases which had lack of male involvement resulted in some complications and C-section deliveries. The observation of the findings reveals there has been increased awareness levels on maternal health part among couples which could be linked to continous efforts of sensitization by the government.

Nuclear families had better indicators of male involvement in most of the cases, as compared to the couples belonging to joint families suggesting the husband is more likely to participate in maternal health services if he belongs to a nuclear family. The study identifies gaps which needs to be addressed , in the view of extraordinary performance of the concept of Mitanins in Chhattisgarh , it was observed that they were not properly prepared to counsel the males, hence the Mitanins are very useful but they need to be properly trained to handle the queries of the males. Similarly the BCC strategies must start focussing on the couples and mens counselling instead of focussing only on women. Interventions related with men's involvement needs to be performed with respect to education, livelihood, poverty. Incentivising male involvement might also help to motivate the working class on larger involvement in maternal and child health programs.

INTRODUCTION

The precursor of the concept of Male involvement in the reproductive health programs was seen in the International conference of population development in Cairo 1994, but in India very few measures have been taken to encourage male involvement in the their partner's reproductive health, Maternal and child mortality in the country is yet to come down and the reasons of the mortality can be seen on various counts. Be it on account of standard delays, or referral, or quality treatment or health consciousness behavior or service delivery pattern. All those aspects are hovering around reproductive health focusing mostly on the women's health and the interventions are planned with women.

The social structure of India subscribes to the norm of keeping men distant from the maternal and child health issues, even though the society is rapidly evolving in its ideologies a large percentage of the rural population find it difficult to understand the importance of the concept of Male involvement in pregnancy and childbirth, they rely on the traditional Dais/Midwives for checkups and delivery, who are often untrained exposing themselves to a range of complications.

There are enough evidences existing in India which suggests that male involvement has a greater net impact on the maternal and child health and can increase the health service utilization as well as outreach of various maternal and child health services being provided. As rightly concluded by (Dudgeon and Inhorn 2004) that men have the capability to influence the health outcomes of Their partners and children "positively" or "Negatively", "Directly" or "Indirectly". This statement fits the Indian scenario due to the high status of a decision maker which is given to an average Indian Male which when directed in an efficient way can actually contribute in reducing the maternal and infant mortality rate in the country which is very much the need of the hour. To fulfil this objective of the study primary data was collected from the eligible couples who fall under the selection criteria of the study i.e expecting couples and couples who have atleast one child of 2 years or less.

Most of the studies have examined the positive effects of men's involvement in maternal and child health, these studies include: (Bhalerao et al. 1984; Carter 2002; Mullany, Becker and Hindin 2007; Singh, Lahiri and Srivastava 2004). The study conducted by Bhalerao et al.(1984) in Mumbai was one of the earliest conducted studies which found that "involving husbands in antenatal care counseling significantly increases the frequency of antenatal care visits, significantly lowers peri-natal mortality, and pays dividends even among uneducated and low socio-economic groups."

A study by Mullany, Becker and Hindin (2007) provided evidence that women tend to understand and utilize the health services and exercise their rights in a better way when they are educated along with their partners. A report by Raju .S and A .Leonard (2000) suggests that "men are interested in becoming more supportive and involved in all reproductive health domains, and that they have reproductive needs of their own which are rarely addressed" and also how "the timing ,location and structure of intervention can encourage or discourage the partner involvement" . Further, in contrast to men who do not participate in antenatal care counselling, men participating in antenatal care counselling tend to know more about family planning, nutrition and health of their wives during pregnancy, and the ways and means of preventing complications during pregnancy, at delivery, or during an abortion. An intervention during prenatal consultations to increase men's involvement in their partners' maternal care increased couples' discussion and use of contraception and improved knowledge about pregnancy and family planning (Varkey et al. 2004).

According to study conducted by M.Carter (2002) among Guatemalan women who had some complications during the pregnancy, considered "type of prenatal care sought and the quality of the familial and marital relationships are important factors ." further he also pointed out the complex nature of male participation as it is not a "singular behaviour" and is subject to influence by various socio-economic, cultural, and gendered norms. Among the studies conducted in India, a study conducted by Abhishek Singh and Faujdar Ram(2009) in Rural Ahmednagar provided a good understanding of the factors which govern the male involvement in their partner's pregnancy and childbirth. This study was an innovative approach to look at male involvement through the lens of 'Gender attitudes' and 'Social Networking.' Further they were also able to substantiate the correlation between male involvement and its positive effects on the overall well being in the health of both mother and child.

According to the NFHS 2005-2006 report of Chhattisgarh state out of 79% of men who claimed that their wives received Antenatal care, Fifty-two percent of men with a child under three said they were present during at least one antenatal check-up received by the child's mother; only one-third were told what to do if the mother had a pregnancy complication, and 10-15 percent were told by a health or family planning worker about specific signs of pregnancy complications. Not all fathers with a child less than three years of age were provided information related to maternal care. Only half (53%) were told about the importance of proper nutrition for the mother during pregnancy and 38 percent were told about the importance of delivering the baby in a health facility. Among fathers whose child was not delivered in a health facility, 58 percent were told about the importance of using a new or unused blade to cut the umbilical cord, 43-44 percent were told about the importance of cleanliness at the time of delivery, and the importance of breastfeeding the baby immediately after birth, and one-fourth were told about keeping the baby warm immediately after birth. The patriarchal nature of society and male domination are the peripheral factors though significant were rarely touched in these reports. If anything can be done that will help yield good results on expected lines by intervening with the male counterparts, it would be an interesting section to delve and also help in designing better strategies. At least 10% of mortality , if curtailed through the greater and effective involvement of Men, it would be a great contribution for the overall efforts. For this to happen a study is necessitated which will basically assess the dimensions of male involvement and the scope for improvement. This will help to redesign the BCC [behavioural change and communication] strategies and also contribute in reducing the maternal and child mortality. The present study is one such attempt to assess the level of male involvement in the partners pregnancy as well as to identify the scope for improving the male involvement thereby reducing the mortality and increasing the coverage of ANC and institutional delivery.

STUDY AIMS AND OBJECTIVES

Study Title : "Male involvement in their partner's pregnancy and childbirth; An Exploratory study in the Bilaspur district of Chhattisgarh state"

This study intends to look at the status of Male involvement in the district of Bilaspur, Chhattisgarh .Male involvement in this study is defined as Men getting involved in decision making, planning of their partners pregnancy, presence in all the ante-natal check-ups, active participation in the counselling process, and support during the pregnancy and Delivery, support which is financial, emotional and in the form of childcare. This study aims to provide an insight into the patterns of men's participation in the pregnancy, childbirth, and its effects on the reproductive health of the women. This will eventually lead to a better understanding of the preferences and perception of men, women and the society they live in about communication between the couple, utilization of health services, and norms dictating the participation of the male partner, which could be addressed in an efficient way further to frame appropriate and relevant policies to encourage male involvement in their partner's pregnancy and childbirth.

The basic study questions attempted to answer in the study are:

- What is the level and affect of involvement of males in their partner's pregnancy?
- How can the males be involved for ensuring safe deliveries and reducing mortality?
- What are the possible methods of involving males in their partner's pregnancy period ?

STUDY APPROACH AND METHODS

The study started on a hypothesis mode wherein it was assumed that 'male involvement has positive effects in maternal and child health' later it took an exploratory orientation while taking references from similar kind of studies to assess the effects of male involvement in the maternal and child health. The purpose of the study has been to gain more familiarity/ insight into the phenomenon of male involvement in the maternal and child health programs and to gain experience that will be helpful in formulating definitive hypothesis for more definite investigation.

Thus the study demanded to adopt a flexible approach like an 'Exploratory research'.

This particular study was performed during the span of one month from 14February till 30 March 2015. A convergent design was framed for the study wherein the intent was to merge concurrent quantitative and qualitative data to address the study aims and objectives, by using a mixed methods research methodology. The interview schedule was designed such that it captured essential information in a quantitative manner while also giving an opportunity to engage the respondents in an 'in-depth conversation' for certain sections of the questionnaires. Thus a semi-structured questionnaire was designed for this purpose. The same study tool was used for Men and women. They were interviewed face-to-face and for each respondent the study collected information on age, years of marriage, number of living children, status of pregnancy, occupation, educational status, type of family. The questionnaire also collected information from the men and women on their awareness on reproductive health behavior, knowledge of immunization schedule, institutional delivery, birth planning, planning of pregnancy, men's willingness to participate in the ANC ,delivery and PNC checkups, decision making , support to the partner in terms of financial, emotional and in childcare, which provide various indicators of men's involvement in their partner's pregnancy and childbirth. The questionnaire comprises of primarily closed ended questions, and also certain open ended questions regarding problems and inconvenience faced by the couple specially the male partner to get involved in the ANC, delivery and PNC checkups. Male involvement during the delivery in this study is defined as male partner being present in the institution at the time of delivery.

SAMPLING PATTERN

The study has been conducted in the Bilaspur district in the Indian state of Chhattisgarh. Bilaspur, being the second largest city after the capital city of Raipur, hosts a population of 331,030 according to 2011 census. The health care needs of the people of Bilaspur are catered by various government and private institutions. The 'District hospital' of Bilaspur was chosen for the study due to its favourable location which hosts patients coming in from nearby villages and from the lower socio economic background. District Hospital provided an ideal setting to understand the perception of the respondents regarding the facilities provided by the government for maternal and child health programs, it also provided a chance to observe the 'social construct' of the respondents and the kind of support they derive from them as almost all the respondents had their relatives and family members with them at the time of admission and delivery.

The study sample was restricted to couples who were expecting and parents of children less than 2 years. 'Random stratified sampling' was opted for the study, with 18 couples interviewed were couples who have had delivery and were admitted in the 'District hospital of Bilaspur'. The rest of the respondents belonged to Three different Anganwadi centres located in the distant areas of Bilaspur covering three different localities of 'village Sarkanda', 'Yadav Muhalla'(Talapara), 'Badhwapara'. These Anganwadi centres were chosen according to convenience. Data collection was also performed by conducting 'household couples interviews', after obtaining their address from the Anganwadi centres, since getting the couples to interview together was pivotal for the study. This also opened gates for counselling the couples in terms of Birth planning, Ante-natal check-ups, Post-natal check-ups, Exclusive breast feeding, Immunization of the child, and other important issues related to maternal and child health. The sample size was 50 eligible couples of the aforementioned selection criteria, and the sample divide was in between couples those who are expecting and parents of children less than or of 2 years of age. During data collection preference was being given to such couples who have had a delivery, because such couples will help to capture all the nuances of pregnancy and childbirth, till the immunization of the child. Thus the sample had 12 expecting couples who belonged to Anganwadi centres, while the rest 38 couples had delivery, or were parents of atleast one child of or less than 2 years of age. Out of these 38 couples 18 were from the District hospital while the rest were those couples who utilized the services of Anganwadi centres. The inclusion criteria of the study involves any pregnant women or parents of a child less than or of 2 years, who have been utilizing the Maternal and child health Facilities of the District hospital as well as the Anganwadi centres. The exclusion criteria involves women who has been admitted to the hospital suffering a miscarriage or have a stillbirth situation, and parents of children of age more than 2 years .

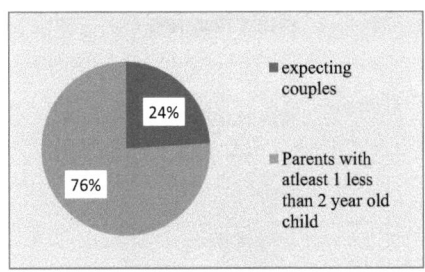

Fig:1 Pie chart showing the percentages of sample taken from 4 different locations.

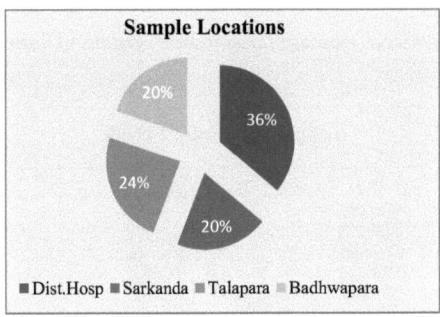

Fig: 2= Pie chart showing the sample break up.

STUDY FINDINGS

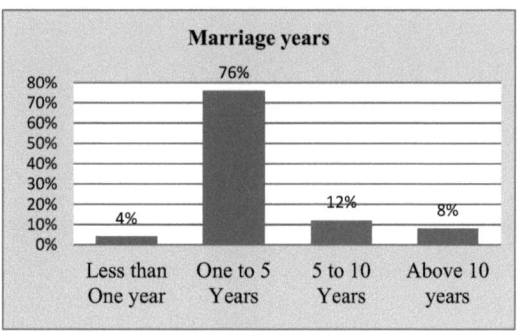

Fig.3: Bar graph showing Years of marriage range from 11 months to 7 years.

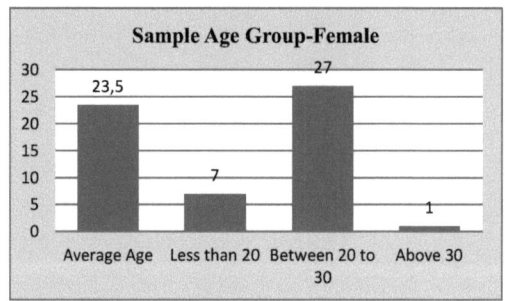

Fig: 4= Bar graph showing sample considered for the study are in the age group of 19 to 34 in females (Average age-23.52).

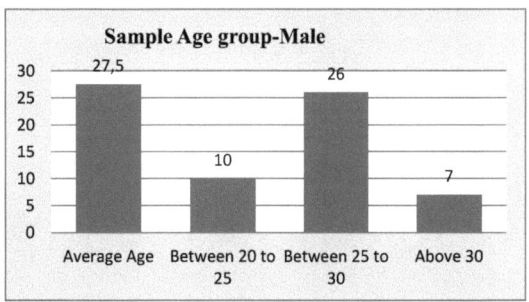

Fig: 5= Bar graph showing Male age group- 22 to 36 (Average age group - 27.56)

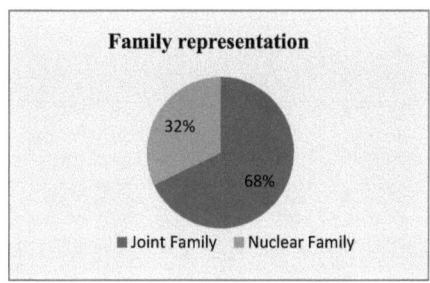

Fig: 6 = Pie chart representing 16 nuclear families and 34 joint families.

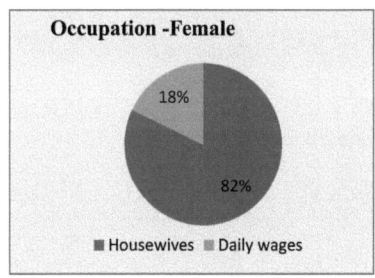

Fig: 7= Pie chart representing Occupation of women – 41 house wife and 4 daily labor.

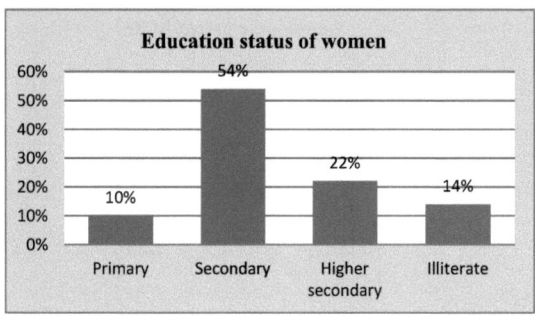

Fig: 8= Bar graph representing the education status of women (Education status – 5 primary, 27 secondary, 11 higher secondary, 7 illiterate).

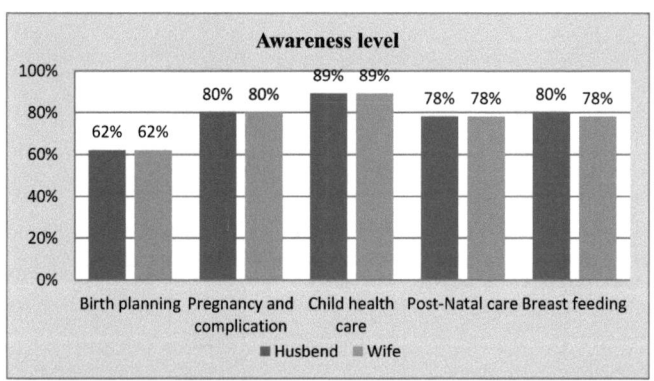

Fig : 9= Awareness levels of both wife and husband about pregnancy and complications, birth planning, child health care, post natal care, exclusive breast feeding.

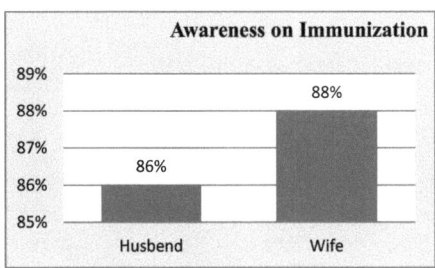

Fig: 10= Bar chart showing levels of awareness between wife and husband about immunization.

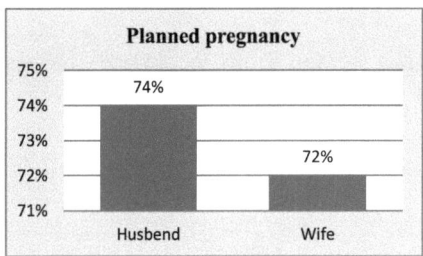

Fig: 11= Bar chart showing levels of awareness about planned pregnancy.

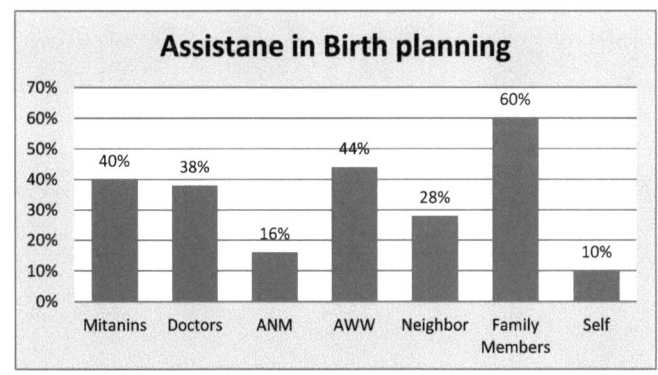

Fig: 12= Bar chart showing assistance received by the couples during birth planning by

Mitanins ,Doctors, Auxillary nurse midwife, Anganwadi worker, Neighbours, Family members, self assistance.

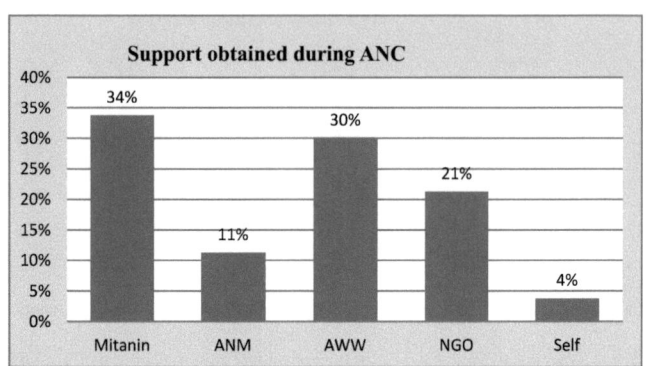

Fig: 13= Bar chart showing assistance received by the couples during Antenatal checkups by Mitanins , Auxillary nurse midwife, Anganwadi worker, NGO, self assistance.

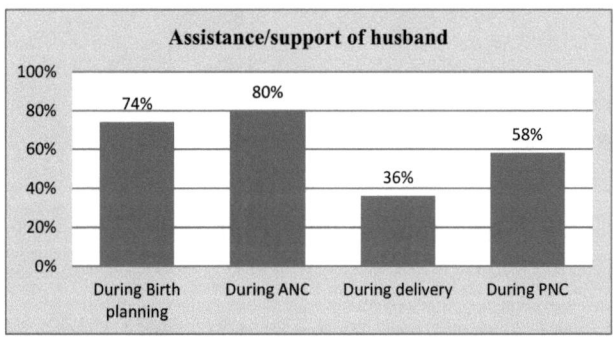

Fig: 14= Bar chart showing assistance given by husband during birth planning, ANC, delivery, PNC.

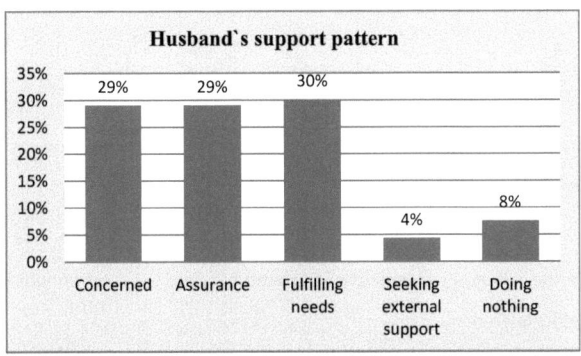

Fig: 15= Bart chart representing husband's support pattern in terms of concern, assurance, fulfilling needs, seeking external support, doing nothing.

STUDY ANALYSIS

IMPORTANT OBSERVATIONS

To perform the study analysis the help of expertise were taken for Data filteration, Indicator analysis, to find out linkages of issues, to understand impact and influence of government schemes and social determinants of health, which led to propose following observations;

- All the cases where there is no involvement of husband resulted in C-section which proves that male involvement as significance.
- 80% of women to whom husband`s contribution are nil are pertaining to Joint families. This indicates that husband`s involvement can increase the decision making power of women.
- Nuclear families have proved better in terms of overall results .
- In the case of joint families it appeared in the analysis that the decision making power of women is comparatively lower. This is an area to concentrate more.
- In more than 30% cases it was observed that the husbands are taking little interest on the child health care especially on hygiene, immunization, malnourishment etc.
- The observation of the findings reveals that there is maximum involvement of husband in most of the cases and the outcome has been encouraging.
- There is certainly an increased awareness level on the maternal health part amongst the couple. This indicates that the government efforts of sensitization has really worked.
- In terms of making of a birth plan, ideally the ANM who is very close to the people should be guiding them largely, however the observation reveals that the contribution of ANM is very marginal. Further the contribution of AWW and Mitanins are very encouraging.
- The observation reveals that most of the cases have very good results as expected and there is large involvement of the males. This could be on account of the urban influence and matured district facilities because Bilaspur is a medically advanced district in the state where there are three big hospitals and it has its urban dynamics. Had the sample been collected from the rural areas the findings would not have been that encouraging. Secondly majority of the couples are educated having largest chunk on higher secondary cadre. There is little percentage of illiterates in the sample.
- The involvement of husband is found at every level and the percentage is sizable beyond the expectations.

- Another important observation includes that the good performance cases are mostly couples with more than five years of marriage age.
- There are still some instances of early marriages and spacing between children are less than three years that resulted into c-sections or complications.
- Already there is a small percentage of males who are capable of making birth plan without seeking any help from others . They are the potential stakeholders in the community.
- The majority of the sample are found in Housewife sections . They have some avenues and no external pressure of economic improvement. However the results of daily workers have the problem of sparing time for the care in pregnancy. Poverty has cascading effect on the health.
- The study reveals that 70% of couples have made birth planning and in 80% of the cases the husband assisted wife in getting ANC checkups.
- Other significant observations include: Only in 36% of cases, the husband was present during the delivery and provided moral and other support to the women. In 58% of cases, the husband made his presence felt to the women during PNC. In 58% of cases the pregnant women suffer from emotional instability. In 32% of cases the husband did not contribute in child care.

There have been certain problems which were also observed redundantly among the couples when questioned about the reasons behind the male partner not being able to participate in the ANC checkups and delivery of their wives. These responses were subjected to domain analysis to capture patterned responses of couples regarding who had certain problems availing healthcare. Thus Domains like factors influencing male involvement , Awareness, Concerns, Health service quality were developed, which were further split into sub-categories each. The relations between the Domains and sub categories revealed certain issues which explains resons for certains men to not get involved in ANCs. There has been no interaction or less interaction between Men and health workers like Mitanins, AWWs, ANMs due to lack of training in these health workers to interact with men. Thus the transmission of information to the men via these health workers is absent resulting in ambiguous perception of men regarding essential Health knowledge. Mostly husband chose to send the mitanins or the mother in law with their wives for checkups. Some couples voiced their hesitations to opt for institutional delivery due to the infamous behavior of the 'uncooperative hospital staff referring to certain instances of violence, bribery, verbal abuse from the part of the hospital staff and other health workers. Hygiene concerns were raised repeatedly by the women admitted in the District hospitals after their delivery, while the men complained about unsatisfactory arrangements of accommodation as most of them hailed from nearby villages and had nowhere to stay in the hospital forced to sleep in the corridors of the Maternity ward.

Issues regarding the neglect of the hospital administration while utilizing their 'smart cards' which allows a below poverty line household to avail cashless health care, provide them with choices,and saves them falling prey to corrupt practices under

' Rashtriya Swasthya Bima Yojana'.

STUDY SUGGESTIONS & CONCLUSION

A lengthy brainstorming session led the investigators to arrive at following conclusions:

- The few males need to be made as the stakeholders in the BCC strategy.
- The counselling and awareness should focus on the couples instead of females.
- The existing BCC efforts are focussing only on the women instead the male group counselling should be initiated.
- The Mitanins are very useful but they need to be properly trained to handle the querries of the males
- The joint families need to be line-listed and approached individually for counselling
- The education need to be promoted for women so that they can handle things.
- The child health care needs to be percolated at communities especially in the male groups.
- The ANM should be more involved in the male involvement drives
- The existing service delivery and BCC strategies need to be revised and it has to be made subject and target oriented instead of making a uniform IEC activities
- Convergence efforts at all levels need to be made in terms of implementing the programmes and activities and education, poverty and livelihood be considered and they are social determinants of health.
- Special incentives for males be provisioned for complete care taking that will motivate them for larger involvement amongst the daily working class.
- The incentive provisions made for institutional delivery be linked with mandatory husband`s presence during the delivery and PNC

CONCLUSION

Undertaking the study is a unique experience for students like us as it gives us exposure to the reality as well as helping to understand the difference between theory and practical. Added to this the task gives us the exposure of study interventions and way it is observed with analysis. The design and application of study tools and assessing the findings are enriching to our experience.

LIMITATIONS

The location for the study were initially selected as the two hospitals that were District hospital and Chhattisgarh institute of Medical sciences. Thus the sample selected was not representative of entire Bilaspur district. However data could not be collected from Chhattisgarh institute of Medical sciences due to unavoidable issues related to obtaining permission for conducting the interviews in the Gynacology department of the Hospital, as the permission letter from the medical superintendent which was dully submitted for the IEC clearance only allowed to conduct interviews but did not address to the Dean of the Gynacology department of the medical college. Thus the study covers only the patients from the district hospital as well as three different Anganwadi centres of Bilaspur district.

The number of pregnant women is comparatively less than the women who have had delivery and couples have a child less than 2 years, of age because preference was given more to couples who have had delivery and are the parents of atleast one child of 2 years or less.The indicators of male involvement during the delivery is only reflective of the fact that male partner has to be present in the institution during and after the delivery but not inside the operation theatre during the childbirth. Men being present during the delivery is a concept which is mostly seen in the metropolitans and only in certain corporate hospitals where such choice is available for men to opt. Whereas in a setting like Chhattisgarh men are not entertained during the time of delivery. In effect nobody except for the staff is allowed to be present during the delivery. Thus indicators of men being present during the delivery has not been included in the study as it is assumed that such indicators will not exist in the particular location.

The observation reveals that most of the cases have very good results as expected and there is large involvement of the males. This could be on account of the urban influence and matured district facilities because Bilaspur is a medically advanced district in the state where there are three big hospitals and it has its urban dynamics. Had the sample been collected from the rural areas the findings would not have been that encouraging

REFERENCES

1.   Abhishek Singh, Faujdar Ram. Men's Involvement during Pregnancy and Childbirth: Evidence from Rural Ahmadnagar, India. Population Review. 2009.

2.   Pulerwitz J, Barker G. Measuring Attitudes toward Gender Norms among Young Men in Brazil: Development and Psychometric Evaluation of the GEM Scale. Men and Masculinities. 2007. p. 322–38.

3.   Bhalerao VR, Galwankar M, Kowli SS, Kumar R, Chaturvedi RM. Contribution of the education of the prospective fathers to the success of maternal health care programme. J Postgrad Med. 1984;30(1):10–2.

4.   Carter MW. "Because he loves me": Husbands' involvement in maternal health in Guatemala. Culture, Health & Sexuality. 2002. p. 259–79.

5.   CONNELL RW. Masculinities and Globalization. Men and Masculinities. 1998. p. 3–23.

6.   Mullany BC, Lakhey B, Shrestha D, Hindin MJ, Becker S. Impact of husbands' participation in antenatal health education services on maternal health knowledge. J Nepal Med Assoc. 2009;48(173):28–34.

7.   Dudgeon MR, Inhorn MC. Men's influences on women's reproductive health: medical anthropological perspectives. Soc Sci Med [Internet]. 2004;59(7):1379–95. Available from: http://www.ncbi.nlm.nih.gov/pubmed/15246168

8.   Mullany BC, Becker S, Hindin MJ. The impact of including husbands in antenatal health education services on maternal health practices in urban Nepal: Results from a randomized controlled trial. Health Educ Res. 2007;22(2):166–76.

9.   India. Department of family health and welfare. National family Health survey;2005-2006.

10. Mendeley [computer program]. Version 1.13.8. Australia: Elsevier; 2013.

ANNEXURES

The questionnaire used in the study is as follows,

Demographic Details:

Name:

- Partner's Name:

Q1) Age:

- partner's age:

Q2) Years of marriage:

Q3) the number and age of children living:

Q4) status of pregnancy:

Q5) Occupation :   5A) Partner's Occupation:

- Agriculture   Agriculture
- Business   Business
- Service   Service
- other(specify)   other(specify)

Q6) Family Type:

- Nuclear
- Non-nuclear

Q7) Education: 7A) Partner's education:

- primary   primary (1)
- >primary<high school   >primary<high school(2)
- More than High School   more than High School (3)
- uneducated   uneducated (4)

Address / Phone:

Awareness

Q8) Do you have information about the following ?:

Respondent: partner:

8A • Birth Planning

8B • pregnancy, childbirth, and about their complications.

8C •women require more care during pregnancy and childbirth.

8D • women need special care after delivery. (Post-natal care)

8E • Children should receive exclusive breastfeeding.

Q9)Are you aware of infant's immunization schedule? (Female and male)

Respondent :   partner:

- Yes
- No

Q10) Where did you/your wife have/had your delivery? / If pregnant then where do you intend to have the delivery?

- Institution
- House / midwife-assisted

male involvement in birth planning:

Q11) was your/your wife's pregnancy planned?

RESPONDENT: PARTNER

- Yes
- No

Q12) did you make a birth plan after pregnancy?

RESPONDENT :   PARTNER:

- Yes (1)
- No (0)

12A) If No, then why ?

- Nobody told about birth planning
- it was not necessary
- Other. ....

12B) If Yes, then who assisted you in birth-planning?

RESPONDENT: PARTNER:

- mitninn
- doctor
- ANM
- Anganwadi Worker
- Neighbour
- Family member
- self decision

Q13) Did you encounter any difficulties during birth planning?

- Yes
- No

13A) If Yes then, what are they?

....

Male involvement in antenatal checkups

Q14) Does your husband accompany you/do you accompany your wife to the Antenatal checkups?

Respondent :   Partner:

- Yes
- No

14A) If yes then, where did you get this information about ANC?

Respondent: partner:

- Mitanin
- ANM
- Anganwadi Worker
- Institution(hospital)
- Self Decision
- Other (SPECIFY)………………………………………………………………………………………………….

Q15) How many Antenatal checkups have you attended till now?

.RESPONDENT…………………………………………PARTNER………………………………………….

Q16) If Yes then do you find it convenient to attend ANC checkups with your wife?/Does your husband find it convenient to attend ANC checkups with you?

Respondent: partner:

- Yes
- No

16A) If No, specify the reason 'why not'?
………

Male involvement in Delivery

Q17) What was the nature of your delivery?

Respondent: Partner:

- -normal
- -operation

17A) Was your husband present during delivery(in the hospital) ?

RESPONDENT   PARTNER

- Yes
- No

Q18) Did you have any problems during delivery ?

RESPONDENT   PARTNER

- Yes (1)
- -No (0)

18A) If so, tell about these issues

....

Men's involvement after deliver

Q19) Do you know about Post natal checkups?

RESPONDANT: PARTNER:

- Yes
- No

19A) If Yes then , what happens in PNC checkups?

....

Q20) Do you participate in all the PNC checkups with your wife and children? Does your husband attend all the PNC checkups with you?

RESPONDANT   PARTNER

- Yes
- No

20A) If No then tell the reason

....

20B) If Yes, then do you find it convenient to attend the PNCs with your wife?

RESPONDANT :   PARTNER:

- Yes
- No

20B1) if No then, tell about your discomfort?

....

Q21) Did you have any problems during your PNC checkups?

RESPONDENT :   PARTNER:

- Yes
- No

21A) If yes then, tell about these issues.

....

Encouragement:

Q22) How many people assisted you and your wife during pregnancy, checkups, delivery and child's immunization?

RESPONDENT: PARTNER:

- Mitanin

- Neighbours
- Family members
- Doctor
- ANM
- AWW
- None Of the above

Assistence to the wife (Emotional support)

Q23) Did you/your wife suffer from emotional instability and insecurities any time during the pregnancy? (

RESPONDENT :   PARTNER:

- Yes
- No

23A)-If Yes then, how does your husband/you handle such a situation?

RESPONDENT: PARTNER:

- He asks you the reason for the emotional state
- Assures you it will be all right
- Asks you about your needs and fulfils them
- Asks someone else to talk to you
- Does nothing about it
- Other(spcify)……………………………………………………………………

Financial support

Q24) During pregnancy did you get the following things for your wife?

RESPONDENT: PARTNER:

- Medications
- Nutritional supplements
- Desired food items
- Appropriate clothes

- Other ....
- Do nothing

Decision-making capacity

Q25) did your wife have her delivery in an institution/if pregnant , do you intend to have your delivery in an institution?

RESPONDENT: PARTNER:

- Yes
- No

Q26) Who all assisted you right from the birth planning , to ANC checkups ,delivery and post natal checkups?

RESPONDANT: PARTNER:

- Husband
- Wife
- Both the husband and wife
- elders/relatives
- Neighbours
- Mitanin
- Anganwadi Worker
- other.... (Mention the authority of the person).....................

Assistence in childcare

Q27) Do you / does your Husband does following things for the baby?

RESPONDANT: PARTNER:

- taking care of the medical needs and immunization of the child
- nutritional care of the child
- handling the child with hygiene
- doesn't contribute to childcare
- Other ....

<u>**Informed Consent Document for Male involvement in their partner's pregnancy and childbirth study in Bilaspur district of Chhattisgarh.**</u>

<u>**Information Sheet**</u>

Male involvement in this study is defined as Men getting involved in decision making, planning of their partners pregnancy, presence in all the ante-natal check- ups, active participation in the counseling process, and support during the pregnancy and Delivery.

The study is being conducted by the primary investigator named-P Vijeyata Naidu, MPH Batch-1,School of Medical Sciences, University of Hyderabad.

Output of the study will be as follows

> ➢ A complete study report after one month.
> ➢ Report constitutes the findings, scope and suggestions to bridge the gap.
> ➢ Dissemination of study findings at appropriate level.

You are invited to participate in the above mentioned study. As a part of this study you will be asked questions on your family details, household details, education, employment and standard of living details, births, deaths, pregnancy, childbirth, details for women in the 15-49 years age group, level of awareness among both men and women about the health care services, feasibility and utilization of such services and your level of satisfaction regarding the services available to encourage Male involvement in the maternal health care.

Answering these questions will take about 30 minutes to 1 hour of your time. You will be approached once for completing the questionnaire and subsequently the field workers may approach you for doubts and clarifications if needed.

There are no major risks for you by participating in this survey. By participating in this study, you will help the investigators to identify scope for improving the male involvement thereby reducing the mortality and increasing the coverage of ANC and institutional delivery and to understand the gaps and the suggestions to facilitate male involvement in maternal healthcare.There will not be any monetary or material compensation for you for participating in the survey.

The information obtained from you may be used for analysis, development of BCC strategies and publication in scientific journals. All information collected from you will be kept confidential. No personal identifying information will be revealed to anyone.

Participation in this study is entirely voluntary. You may withdraw from the study or refuse to participate at any point. In case you have any doubts or question you should ask these to the person who is administering this questionnaire to you. You can decide on participating after all your doubts and questions have been answered to your satisfaction.

Consent Form

Participant's Initials: _____ Participant's Name: _____

Date of Birth / Age:_____

(i) I confirm that I have read and understood the information sheet dated _____ for the above study and have had the opportunity to ask questions. OR I confirm that the information sheet has been read out to me to my understanding and I have had the opportunity to ask questions. [ ]

(ii) I understand that my participation in the study is voluntary and that I am free to withdraw at any time, without giving any reason, without my medical care or legal rights being affected. [ ]

(iii) I understand that the Sponsor of the survey, others working for the survey, the Ethics Committee and the regulatory authorities will not need my permission to look at my records both in respect of the current study and any further research that may be conducted in relation to it, even if I withdraw from the trial. I agree to this access. However, I understand that my identity will not be revealed in any information released to third parties or published. [ ]

(iv) I agree not to restrict the use of any data or results that arise from this study provided such a use is only for scientific purpose(s) [ ]

(v) I agree to take part in the above survey. [ ]

Signature of the Participant or Legally Acceptable Representative:_____

Date: _____/_____/_____

Signatory's Name: _____

Signature of the Investigator: _____

Date: _____ / _____ / _____

Study Investigator's Name: _____

Signature of Impartial Witness: _____

Date: _____ / _____ / _____

Name of the Witness: _____

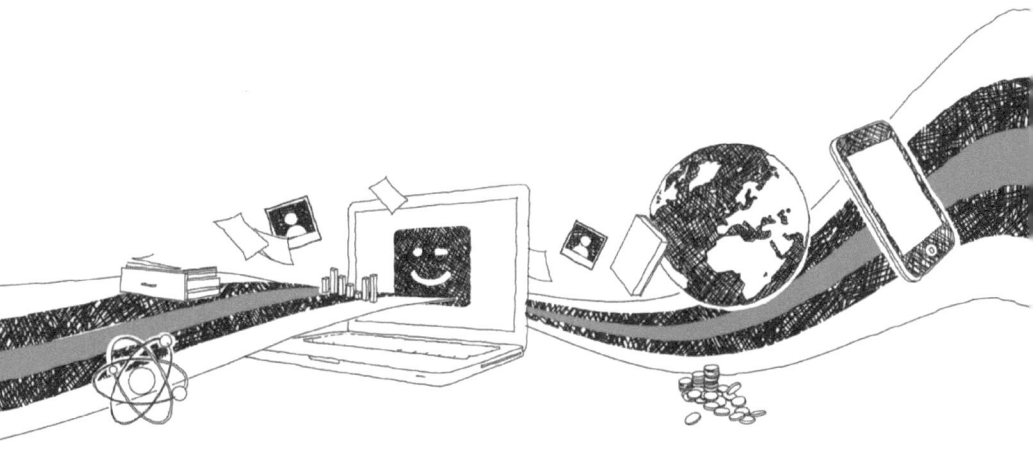
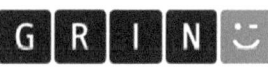